This Weight Loss Tracker Belongs To:

Jennifer Anthony

Jul 25

Help us grow, please review and rate.
Oh La La Planners and Organizers

Motivation:

_____

_____

_____

_____

_____

_____

_____

_____

_____

Action Plan

_____

_____

_____

_____

_____

_____

_____

_____

_____

Focus:

_____

_____

_____

_____

_____

_____

Week Of:................................

New Habits To Built

Old Habits To Cut

Measurements:
BUST:

WAIST:

HIPS:

CHEST:

THIGHS:

ARM:

This Week's Goal:

Weekly Difficulties:

Weekly Successes:

This Week's Weight Loss:

Total Weight Loss:

DATE...................................

Fasting Day? Yes No   Feeding Window: 2 4 6 8 10 12

Meals:	Time:	Calories:

Water Intake: 🥛🥛🥛🥛🥛🥛🥛🥛🥛   Supplements: 💊💊💊

Exercise	Time/Distance/Steps/Sets	Calories/Goal Achieved?

My Notes:
_____
_____
_____

Overall Feelings:	Awful	Not Good	OK	Great	Awesome
Energy:	😖	😐	🙂	😁	😍
Nutrition:	😖	😐	🙂	😁	😍
Exercise:	😖	😐	🙂	😁	😍

Sleep Time:................   Weight AM:................   Weight AM:................

DATE.....................

Fasting Day? Yes No   Feeding Window: 2 4 6 8 10 12

Meals:		Time:	Calories:

Water Intake: 🥤🥤🥤🥤🥤🥤🥤🥤🥤🥤   Supplements: 💊💊💊

Exercise	Time/Distance/Steps/Sets	Calories/Goal Achieved?

My Notes:

Overall Feelings:	Awful	Not Good	OK	Great	Awesome
Energy:	😖	😐	🙂	😁	😍
Nutrition:	😖	😐	🙂	😁	😍
Exercise:	😖	😐	🙂	😁	😍

Sleep Time:...........   Weight AM:...........   Weight AM:...........

DATE...........................

Fasting Day? Yes No   Feeding Window: 2 4 6 8 10 12

Meals:	Time:	Calories:

Water Intake: ☐ ☐ ☐ ☐ ☐ ☐ ☐ ☐ ☐   Supplements: ◯ ◯ ◯

Exercise	Time/Distance/Steps/Sets	Calories/Goal Achieved?

My Notes:

Overall Feelings:	Awful	Not Good	OK	Great	Awesome
Energy:	😖	😐	🙂	😁	😍
Nutrition:	😖	😐	🙂	😁	😍
Exercise:	😖	😐	🙂	😁	😍

Sleep Time:...........   Weight AM:...............   Weight AM:...............

DATE......................................

Fasting Day? Yes No   Feeding Window: 2 4 6 8 10 12

Meals:	Time:	Calories:

Water Intake: ▯▯▯▯▯▯▯▯▯▯   Supplements: ⬭ ⬭ ⬭

Exercise	Time/Distance/Steps/Sets	Calories/Goal Achieved?

My Notes:
_____
_____
_____

Overall Feelings:	Awful	Not Good	OK	Great	Awesome
Energy:	😖	😐	🙂	😁	😍
Nutrition:	😖	😐	🙂	😁	😍
Exercise:	😖	😐	🙂	😁	😍

Sleep Time:............   Weight AM:............   Weight AM:............

DATE................................

Fasting Day? Yes No   Feeding Window: 2 4 6 8 10 12

Meals:		Time:	Calories:

Water Intake: ▯ ▯ ▯ ▯ ▯ ▯ ▯ ▯ ▯ ▯   Supplements: ◯ ◯ ◯

Exercise	Time/Distance/Steps/Sets	Calories/Goal Achieved?

My Notes: _____
_____
_____
_____

Overall Feelings:	Awful	Not Good	OK	Great	Awesome
Energy:	😖	😐	🙂	😁	😊
Nutrition:	😖	😐	🙂	😁	😊
Exercise:	😖	😐	🙂	😁	😊

Sleep Time:...............   Weight AM:................   Weight AM:................

DATE......................

Fasting Day? Yes No   Feeding Window: 2 4 6 8 10 12

Meals:	Time:	Calories:

Water Intake: 🥛🥛🥛🥛🥛🥛🥛🥛🥛🥛 Supplements: 💊💊💊

Exercise	Time/Distance/Steps/Sets	Calories/Goal Achieved?

My Notes:
_____
_____
_____

Overall Feelings:	Awful	Not Good	OK	Great	Awesome
Energy:	😖	😐	🙂	😁	😊
Nutrition:	😖	😐	🙂	😁	😊
Exercise:	😖	😐	🙂	😁	😊

Sleep Time:..............   Weight AM:..............   Weight AM:..............

DATE......................................

Fasting Day? Yes No   Feeding Window: 2 4 6 8 10 12

Meals:	Time:	Calories:

Water Intake: ☐ ☐ ☐ ☐ ☐ ☐ ☐ ☐ ☐   Supplements: ⊘ ⊘ ⊘

Exercise	Time/Distance/Steps/Sets	Calories/Goal Achieved?

My Notes:
_____
_____
_____

Overall Feelings:	Awful	Not Good	OK	Great	Awesome
Energy:	😖	😐	🙂	😁	😊
Nutrition:	😖	😐	🙂	😁	😊
Exercise:	😖	😐	🙂	😁	😊

Sleep Time:.............   Weight AM:.............   Weight AM:.............

Week Of:.......................

New Habits To Built

Old Habits To Cut

Measurements:
BUST:

WAIST:

HIPS:

CHEST:

THIGHS:

ARM:

This Week's Goal:

Weekly Difficulties:

Weekly Successes:

This Week's Weight Loss:

Total Weight Loss:

DATE..............................

Fasting Day? Yes No   Feeding Window: 2 4 6 8 10 12

Meals:	Time:	Calories:

Water Intake: ☐ ☐ ☐ ☐ ☐ ☐ ☐ ☐ ☐ ☐   Supplements: ◯ ◯ ◯

Exercise	Time/Distance/Steps/Sets	Calories/Goal Achieved?

My Notes:

Overall Feelings:	Awful	Not Good	OK	Great	Awesome
Energy:	😖	😐	🙂	😁	😍
Nutrition:	😖	😐	🙂	😁	😍
Exercise:	😖	😐	🙂	😁	😍

Sleep Time:..............   Weight AM:................   Weight AM:................

DATE..

Fasting Day? Yes No   Feeding Window: 2 4 6 8 10 12

Meals:		Time:	Calories:

Water Intake: 🥛🥛🥛🥛🥛🥛🥛🥛🥛🥛   Supplements: 💊💊💊

Exercise	Time/Distance/Steps/Sets	Calories/Goal Achieved?

My Notes:
_____
_____
_____

Overall Feelings:	Awful	Not Good	OK	Great	Awesome
Energy:	😖	😐	🙂	😁	😍
Nutrition:	😖	😐	🙂	😁	😍
Exercise:	😖	😐	🙂	😁	😍

Sleep Time:............   Weight AM:............   Weight AM:............

DATE...........................

Fasting Day? Yes No   Feeding Window: 2 4 6 8 10 12

Meals:	Time:	Calories:

Water Intake: ▯ ▯ ▯ ▯ ▯ ▯ ▯ ▯ ▯ ▯   Supplements: ⬭ ⬭ ⬭

Exercise	Time/Distance/Steps/Sets	Calories/Goal Achieved?

My Notes:
_____
_____
_____

Overall Feelings:	Awful	Not Good	OK	Great	Awesome
Energy:	😖	😐	🙂	😁	😍
Nutrition:	😖	😐	🙂	😁	😍
Exercise:	😖	😐	🙂	😁	😍

Sleep Time:...........   Weight AM:...............   Weight AM:...............

DATE..

Fasting Day? Yes No   Feeding Window: 2 4 6 8 10 12

Meals:	Time:	Calories:

Water Intake: 🥛🥛🥛🥛🥛🥛🥛🥛🥛🥛   Supplements: 💊💊💊

Exercise	Time/Distance/Steps/Sets	Calories/Goal Achieved?

My Notes:
_____
_____
_____

Overall Feelings:	Awful	Not Good	OK	Great	Awesome
Energy:	😣	😐	🙂	😁	😍
Nutrition:	😣	😐	🙂	😁	😍
Exercise:	😣	😐	🙂	😁	😍

Sleep Time:..............   Weight AM:..............   Weight AM:..............

DATE..............................

Fasting Day? Yes No   Feeding Window: 2 4 6 8 10 12

Meals:	Time:	Calories:

Water Intake: 🥛🥛🥛🥛🥛🥛🥛🥛🥛🥛   Supplements: 💊💊💊

Exercise	Time/Distance/Steps/Sets	Calories/Goal Achieved?

My Notes:
_____
_____
_____

Overall Feelings:	Awful	Not Good	OK	Great	Awesome
Energy:	😣	😐	🙂	😁	😍
Nutrition:	😣	😐	🙂	😁	😍
Exercise:	😣	😐	🙂	😁	😍

Sleep Time:..............   Weight AM:..............   Weight AM:..............

DATE............................

Fasting Day? Yes No   Feeding Window: 2 4 6 8 10 12

Meals:		Time:	Calories:

Water Intake: 🥛🥛🥛🥛🥛🥛🥛🥛🥛🥛   Supplements: 💊 💊 💊

Exercise	Time/Distance/Steps/Sets	Calories/Goal Achieved?

My Notes:
_____
_____
_____

Overall Feelings:	Awful	Not Good	OK	Great	Awesome
Energy:	😣	😐	🙂	😁	😍
Nutrition:	😣	😐	🙂	😁	😍
Exercise:	😣	😐	🙂	😁	😍

Sleep Time:............   Weight AM:............   Weight AM:............

DATE................................

Fasting Day? Yes No   Feeding Window: 2 4 6 8 10 12

Meals:	Time:	Calories:

Water Intake: 🥛🥛🥛🥛🥛🥛🥛🥛🥛🥛   Supplements: 💊💊💊

Exercise	Time/Distance/Steps/Sets	Calories/Goal Achieved?

My Notes:
_____
_____
_____

Overall Feelings:	Awful	Not Good	OK	Great	Awesome
Energy:	😖	😐	🙂	😁	😍
Nutrition:	😖	😐	🙂	😁	😍
Exercise:	😖	😐	🙂	😁	😍

Sleep Time:...............   Weight AM:...............   Weight AM:...............

Week Of:................................

New Habits To Built

Old Habits To Cut

Measurements:
BUST:

WAIST:

HIPS:

CHEST:

THIGHS:

ARM:

This Week's Goal:

Weekly Difficulties:

Weekly Successes:

This Week's Weight Loss:

Total Weight Loss:

DATE................................

Fasting Day? Yes No   Feeding Window: 2 4 6 8 10 12

Meals:	Time:	Calories:

Water Intake: 🥛🥛🥛🥛🥛🥛🥛🥛🥛   Supplements: 💊💊💊

Exercise	Time/Distance/Steps/Sets	Calories/Goal Achieved?

My Notes:
_____
_____
_____

Overall Feelings:	Awful	Not Good	OK	Great	Awesome
Energy:	😖	😐	🙂	😁	😍
Nutrition:	😖	😐	🙂	😁	😍
Exercise:	😖	😐	🙂	😁	😍

Sleep Time:............   Weight AM:............   Weight AM:............

DATE........................

| Fasting Day? Yes No | | Feeding Window: 2 4 6 8 10 12 |

Meals:		Time:	Calories:

Water Intake: 🥛🥛🥛🥛🥛🥛🥛🥛🥛🥛 Supplements: 💊💊💊

Exercise	Time/Distance/Steps/Sets	Calories/Goal Achieved?

My Notes:

Overall Feelings:	Awful	Not Good	OK	Great	Awesome
Energy:	😖	😐	🙂	😁	😍
Nutrition:	😖	😐	🙂	😁	😍
Exercise:	😖	😐	🙂	😁	😍

Sleep Time:............   Weight AM:............   Weight AM:............

DATE..........................

Fasting Day?   Yes   No   Feeding Window: 2   4   6   8   10   12

Meals:		Time:	Calories:

Water Intake: [glass] [glass] [glass] [glass] [glass] [glass] [glass] [glass] [glass]   Supplements: [pill] [pill] [pill]

Exercise	Time/Distance/Steps/Sets	Calories/Goal Achieved?

My Notes:
_____
_____
_____

Overall Feelings:	Awful	Not Good	OK	Great	Awesome
Energy:	😖	😐	🙂	😁	😊
Nutrition:	😖	😐	🙂	😁	😊
Exercise:	😖	😐	🙂	😁	😊

Sleep Time:..............   Weight AM:..............   Weight AM:..............

DATE...

Fasting Day? Yes No   Feeding Window: 2 4 6 8 10 12

Meals:		Time:	Calories:

Water Intake: [ ] [ ] [ ] [ ] [ ] [ ] [ ] [ ] [ ] [ ]   Supplements: ▱ ▱ ▱

Exercise	Time/Distance/Steps/Sets	Calories/Goal Achieved?

My Notes:
_____
_____
_____

Overall Feelings:	Awful	Not Good	OK	Great	Awesome
Energy:	😖	😐	🙂	😁	😍
Nutrition:	😖	😐	🙂	😁	😍
Exercise:	😖	😐	🙂	😁	😍

Sleep Time:............   Weight AM:............   Weight AM:............

DATE...........................

Fasting Day? Yes No   Feeding Window: 2 4 6 8 10 12

Meals:		Time:	Calories:

Water Intake: 🥛🥛🥛🥛🥛🥛🥛🥛🥛🥛   Supplements: 💊💊💊

Exercise	Time/Distance/Steps/Sets	Calories/Goal Achieved?

My Notes:

Overall Feelings:	Awful	Not Good	OK	Great	Awesome
Energy:	😖	😐	🙂	😁	😍
Nutrition:	😖	😐	🙂	😁	😍
Exercise:	😖	😐	🙂	😁	😍

Sleep Time:...........   Weight AM:..............   Weight AM:..............

DATE.........................

Fasting Day? Yes No   Feeding Window: 2 4 6 8 10 12

Meals:		Time:	Calories:

Water Intake: 🥛🥛🥛🥛🥛🥛🥛🥛🥛🥛   Supplements: 💊💊💊

Exercise	Time/Distance/Steps/Sets	Calories/Goal Achieved?

My Notes:
_____
_____
_____

Overall Feelings:	Awful	Not Good	OK	Great	Awesome
Energy:	😣	😐	🙂	😃	😍
Nutrition:	😣	😐	🙂	😃	😍
Exercise:	😣	😐	🙂	😃	😍

Sleep Time:...............   Weight AM:...............   Weight AM:...............

DATE............................

Fasting Day? Yes No   Feeding Window: 2 4 6 8 10 12

Meals:		Time:	Calories:

Water Intake: ⬜⬜⬜⬜⬜⬜⬜⬜⬜⬜   Supplements: ⬭⬭⬭

Exercise	Time/Distance/Steps/Sets	Calories/Goal Achieved?

My Notes:
_____
_____
_____

Overall Feelings:	Awful	Not Good	OK	Great	Awesome
Energy:	😖	😐	🙂	😁	😍
Nutrition:	😖	😐	🙂	😁	😍
Exercise:	😖	😐	🙂	😁	😍

Sleep Time:............   Weight AM:...............   Weight AM:...............

Week Of:...............................

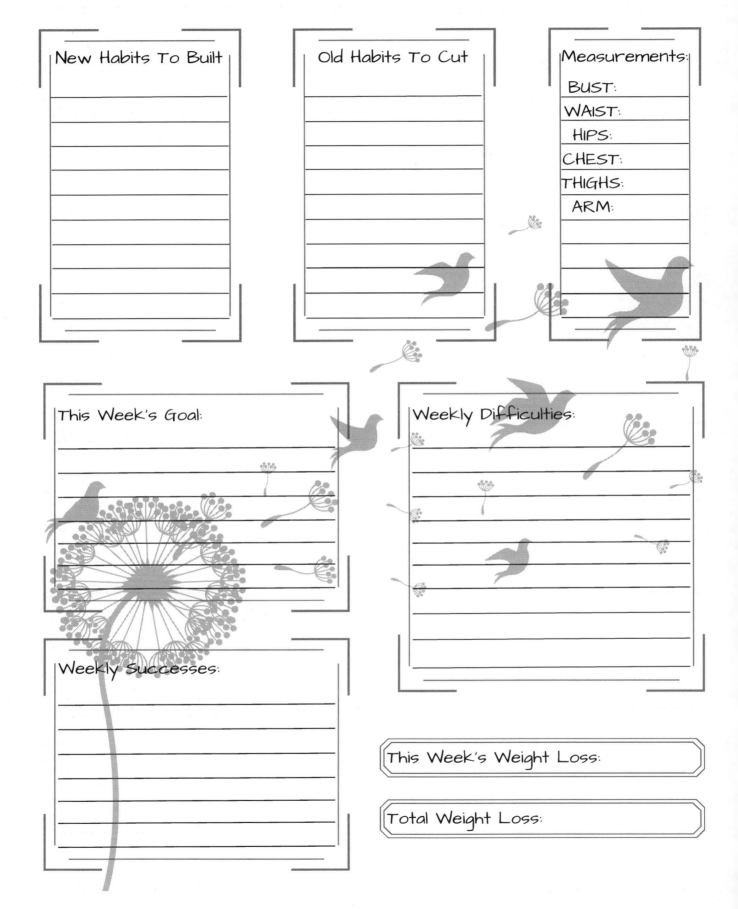

New Habits To Built

Old Habits To Cut

Measurements:
- BUST:
- WAIST:
- HIPS:
- CHEST:
- THIGHS:
- ARM:

This Week's Goal:

Weekly Difficulties:

Weekly Successes:

This Week's Weight Loss:

Total Weight Loss:

DATE............................

Fasting Day? Yes No   Feeding Window: 2 4 6 8 10 12

Meals:	Time:	Calories:

Water Intake: 🥛🥛🥛🥛🥛🥛🥛🥛🥛🥛   Supplements: 💊💊💊

Exercise	Time/Distance/Steps/Sets	Calories/Goal Achieved?

My Notes:

Overall Feelings:	Awful	Not Good	OK	Great	Awesome
Energy:	😣	😐	🙂	😁	😍
Nutrition:	😣	😐	🙂	😁	😍
Exercise:	😣	😐	🙂	😁	😍

Sleep Time:............   Weight AM:...............   Weight AM:...............

DATE..

Fasting Day? Yes No   Feeding Window: 2 4 6 8 10 12

Meals:		Time:	Calories:

Water Intake: 🥛🥛🥛🥛🥛🥛🥛🥛🥛🥛   Supplements: 💊💊💊

Exercise	Time/Distance/Steps/Sets	Calories/Goal Achieved?

My Notes:
_____
_____
_____

Overall Feelings:	Awful	Not Good	OK	Great	Awesome
Energy:	😖	😐	🙂	😁	😍
Nutrition:	😖	😐	🙂	😁	😍
Exercise:	😖	😐	🙂	😁	😍

Sleep Time:............   Weight AM:............   Weight AM:............

DATE..

Fasting Day? Yes No   Feeding Window: 2 4 6 8 10 12

Meals:	Time:	Calories:

Water Intake: ⬜⬜⬜⬜⬜⬜⬜⬜⬜⬜ Supplements: ⬭⬭⬭

Exercise	Time/Distance/Steps/Sets	Calories/Goal Achieved?

My Notes:

Overall Feelings:	Awful	Not Good	OK	Great	Awesome
Energy:	😖	😐	🙂	😁	😍
Nutrition:	😖	😐	🙂	😁	😍
Exercise:	😖	😐	🙂	😁	😍

Sleep Time:............   Weight AM:............   Weight AM:............

DATE............................

Fasting Day? Yes No   Feeding Window: 2 4 6 8 10 12

Meals:		Time:	Calories:

Water Intake: 🥛🥛🥛🥛🥛🥛🥛🥛🥛🥛   Supplements: 💊💊💊

Exercise	Time/Distance/Steps/Sets	Calories/Goal Achieved?

My Notes:
_____
_____
_____

Overall Feelings:	Awful	Not Good	OK	Great	Awesome
Energy:	😣	😐	🙂	😁	😊
Nutrition:	😣	😐	🙂	😁	😊
Exercise:	😣	😐	🙂	😁	😊

Sleep Time:............   Weight AM:............   Weight AM:............

DATE...................................

Fasting Day? Yes No   Feeding Window: 2 4 6 8 10 12

Meals:	Time:	Calories:

Water Intake: 🥛🥛🥛🥛🥛🥛🥛🥛🥛🥛   Supplements: 💊💊💊

Exercise	Time/Distance/Steps/Sets	Calories/Goal Achieved?

My Notes:

Overall Feelings:	Awful	Not Good	OK	Great	Awesome
Energy:					
Nutrition:					
Exercise:					

Sleep Time:................   Weight AM:................   Weight AM:................

DATE................................

Fasting Day? Yes No   Feeding Window: 2 4 6 8 10 12

Meals:		Time:	Calories:

Water Intake: 🥛🥛🥛🥛🥛🥛🥛🥛🥛🥛   Supplements: 💊💊💊

Exercise	Time/Distance/Steps/Sets	Calories/Goal Achieved?

My Notes:
_____
_____
_____

Overall Feelings:	Awful	Not Good	OK	Great	Awesome
Energy:	😖	😐	🙂	😁	😍
Nutrition:	😖	😐	🙂	😁	😍
Exercise:	😖	😐	🙂	😁	😍

Sleep Time:...............   Weight AM:...............   Weight AM:...............

DATE....................

Fasting Day? Yes No   **Feeding Window:** 2 4 6 8 10 12

Meals:		Time:	Calories:

Water Intake: ☐ ☐ ☐ ☐ ☐ ☐ ☐ ☐ ☐ ☐   **Supplements:** ⬭ ⬭ ⬭

Exercise	Time/Distance/Steps/Sets	Calories/Goal Achieved?

My Notes:

Overall Feelings:	Awful	Not Good	OK	Great	Awesome
Energy:	😖	🙂	🙂	😁	😍
Nutrition:	😖	🙂	🙂	😁	😍
Exercise:	😖	🙂	🙂	😁	😍

Sleep Time:............   **Weight AM:**.............   **Weight AM:**.............

Week Of:......................

New Habits To Built

Old Habits To Cut

Measurements:
BUST:

WAIST:

HIPS:

CHEST:

THIGHS:

ARM:

This Week's Goal:

Weekly Difficulties:

Weekly Successes:

This Week's Weight Loss:

Total Weight Loss:

DATE.............................

Fasting Day? Yes No   Feeding Window: 2 4 6 8 10 12

Meals:	Time:	Calories:

Water Intake: ▯ ▯ ▯ ▯ ▯ ▯ ▯ ▯ ▯ ▯   Supplements: ⬭ ⬭ ⬭

Exercise	Time/Distance/Steps/Sets	Calories/Goal Achieved?

My Notes:
_____
_____
_____

Overall Feelings:	Awful	Not Good	OK	Great	Awesome
Energy:	😣	😐	🙂	😁	😍
Nutrition:	😣	😐	🙂	😁	😍
Exercise:	😣	😐	🙂	😁	😍

Sleep Time:............   Weight AM:............   Weight AM:............

DATE...........................

Fasting Day? Yes No   Feeding Window: 2 4 6 8 10 12

Meals:		Time:	Calories:

Water Intake: 🥛🥛🥛🥛🥛🥛🥛🥛🥛🥛   Supplements: 💊💊💊

Exercise	Time/Distance/Steps/Sets	Calories/Goal Achieved?

My Notes:

Overall Feelings:	Awful	Not Good	OK	Great	Awesome
Energy:	😖	😐	🙂	😁	😍
Nutrition:	😖	😐	🙂	😁	😍
Exercise:	😖	😐	🙂	😁	😍

Sleep Time:...............   Weight AM:...............   Weight AM:...............

DATE.............................

Fasting Day? Yes No   Feeding Window: 2 4 6 8 10 12

Meals:	Time:	Calories:

Water Intake: ☐ ☐ ☐ ☐ ☐ ☐ ☐ ☐ ☐ ☐   Supplements: ⬭ ⬭ ⬭

Exercise	Time/Distance/Steps/Sets	Calories/Goal Achieved?

My Notes:
_____
_____
_____

Overall Feelings:	Awful	Not Good	OK	Great	Awesome
Energy:	😖	😐	🙂	😁	😊
Nutrition:	😖	😐	🙂	😁	😊
Exercise:	😖	😐	🙂	😁	😊

Sleep Time:.............   Weight AM:.............   Weight AM:.............

DATE.....................................

Fasting Day? Yes No   Feeding Window: 2 4 6 8 10 12

Meals:	Time:	Calories:

Water Intake: 🥛🥛🥛🥛🥛🥛🥛🥛🥛🥛   Supplements: 💊💊💊

Exercise	Time/Distance/Steps/Sets	Calories/Goal Achieved?

My Notes:
_____
_____
_____

Overall Feelings:	Awful	Not Good	OK	Great	Awesome
Energy:	😖	😐	🙂	😁	😍
Nutrition:	😖	😐	🙂	😁	😍
Exercise:	😖	😐	🙂	😁	😍

Sleep Time:...............   Weight AM:...............   Weight AM:...............

DATE...

Fasting Day? Yes No   Feeding Window: 2 4 6 8 10 12

Meals:		Time:	Calories:

Water Intake: 🥛🥛🥛🥛🥛🥛🥛🥛🥛🥛   Supplements: 💊💊💊

Exercise	Time/Distance/Steps/Sets	Calories/Goal Achieved?

My Notes:
_____
_____
_____

Overall Feelings:	Awful	Not Good	OK	Great	Awesome
Energy:	😖	😐	🙂	😁	😍
Nutrition:	😖	😐	🙂	😁	😍
Exercise:	😖	😐	🙂	😁	😍

Sleep Time:.............   Weight AM:.............   Weight AM:.............

DATE......................................

Fasting Day? Yes No   Feeding Window: 2 4 6 8 10 12

Meals:		Time:	Calories:

Water Intake: 🥛🥛🥛🥛🥛🥛🥛🥛🥛🥛   Supplements: 💊💊💊

Exercise	Time/Distance/Steps/Sets	Calories/Goal Achieved?

My Notes:
_____
_____
_____

Overall Feelings:	Awful	Not Good	OK	Great	Awesome
Energy:	😖	😐	🙂	😁	🥰
Nutrition:	😖	😐	🙂	😁	🥰
Exercise:	😖	😐	🙂	😁	🥰

Sleep Time:...............   Weight AM:...............   Weight AM:...............

DATE...

Fasting Day? Yes No   Feeding Window: 2 4 6 8 10 12

Meals:		Time:	Calories:

Water Intake: [ ][ ][ ][ ][ ][ ][ ][ ][ ]   Supplements: ⬭ ⬭ ⬭

Exercise	Time/Distance/Steps/Sets	Calories/Goal Achieved?

My Notes: _____
_____
_____

Overall Feelings:	Awful	Not Good	OK	Great	Awesome
Energy:	😣	😐	🙂	😁	😍
Nutrition:	😣	😐	🙂	😁	😍
Exercise:	😣	😐	🙂	😁	😍

Sleep Time:................   Weight AM:................   Weight AM:................

Week Of:..

New Habits To Built

Old Habits To Cut

Measurements:
BUST:
WAIST:
HIPS:
CHEST:
THIGHS:
ARM:

This Week's Goal:

Weekly Difficulties:

Weekly Successes:

This Week's Weight Loss:

Total Weight Loss:

DATE................................

Fasting Day? Yes No   **Feeding Window:** 2 4 6 8 10 12

Meals:	Time:	Calories:

Water Intake: ⬜ ⬜ ⬜ ⬜ ⬜ ⬜ ⬜ ⬜ ⬜   **Supplements:** ⬭ ⬭ ⬭

Exercise	Time/Distance/Steps/Sets	Calories/Goal Achieved?

My Notes:

Overall Feelings:	Awful	Not Good	OK	Great	Awesome
Energy:	😖	😐	🙂	😁	😊
Nutrition:	😖	😐	🙂	😁	😊
Exercise:	😖	😐	🙂	😁	😊

Sleep Time:................   Weight AM:................   Weight AM:................

DATE................................

Fasting Day? Yes No   Feeding Window: 2 4 6 8 10 12

Meals:	Time:	Calories:

Water Intake: 🥛🥛🥛🥛🥛🥛🥛🥛🥛🥛   Supplements: 💊💊💊

Exercise	Time/Distance/Steps/Sets	Calories/Goal Achieved?

My Notes:
_____
_____
_____

Overall Feelings:	Awful	Not Good	OK	Great	Awesome
Energy:	😖	😐	🙂	😀	😍
Nutrition:	😖	😐	🙂	😀	😍
Exercise:	😖	😐	🙂	😀	😍

Sleep Time:..............   Weight AM:..............   Weight AM:..............

DATE............................

Fasting Day? Yes No   Feeding Window: 2 4 6 8 10 12

Meals:	Time:	Calories:

Water Intake: ▢ ▢ ▢ ▢ ▢ ▢ ▢ ▢ ▢ ▢   Supplements: ⬭ ⬭ ⬭

Exercise	Time/Distance/Steps/Sets	Calories/Goal Achieved?

My Notes:
_____
_____
_____

Overall Feelings:	Awful	Not Good	OK	Great	Awesome
Energy:	😣	😐	🙂	😁	😊
Nutrition:	😣	😐	🙂	😁	😊
Exercise:	😣	😐	🙂	😁	😊

Sleep Time:............   Weight AM:............   Weight AM:............

DATE................................

Fasting Day? Yes No   Feeding Window: 2 4 6 8 10 12

Meals:	Time:	Calories:

Water Intake: 🥛🥛🥛🥛🥛🥛🥛🥛🥛🥛   Supplements: 💊💊💊

Exercise	Time/Distance/Steps/Sets	Calories/Goal Achieved?

My Notes:

Overall Feelings:	Awful	Not Good	OK	Great	Awesome
Energy:	😖	😐	🙂	😁	😊
Nutrition:	😖	😐	🙂	😁	😊
Exercise:	😖	😐	🙂	😁	😊

Sleep Time:................   Weight AM:................   Weight AM:................

DATE................................

Fasting Day? Yes No   Feeding Window: 2 4 6 8 10 12

Meals:		Time:	Calories:

Water Intake: ▯ ▯ ▯ ▯ ▯ ▯ ▯ ▯ ▯ ▯   Supplements: ⬭ ⬭ ⬭

Exercise	Time/Distance/Steps/Sets	Calories/Goal Achieved?

My Notes:
_____
_____
_____

Overall Feelings:	Awful	Not Good	OK	Great	Awesome
Energy:	😖	😐	🙂	😁	😍
Nutrition:	😖	😐	🙂	😁	😍
Exercise:	😖	😐	🙂	😁	😍

Sleep Time:.............   Weight AM:.............   Weight AM:.............

DATE............................

Fasting Day? Yes No   Feeding Window: 2 4 6 8 10 12

Meals:	Time:	Calories:

Water Intake: [glasses] Supplements: [pills]

Exercise	Time/Distance/Steps/Sets	Calories/Goal Achieved?

My Notes:
_____
_____
_____

Overall Feelings:	Awful	Not Good	OK	Great	Awesome
Energy:	😖	😐	🙂	😁	😍
Nutrition:	😖	😐	🙂	😁	😍
Exercise:	😖	😐	🙂	😁	😍

Sleep Time:............   Weight AM:............   Weight AM:............

DATE....................................

Fasting Day? Yes No   Feeding Window: 2 4 6 8 10 12

Meals:	Time:	Calories:

Water Intake: 🥛🥛🥛🥛🥛🥛🥛🥛🥛🥛   Supplements: 💊💊💊

Exercise	Time/Distance/Steps/Sets	Calories/Goal Achieved?

My Notes:
_____
_____
_____

Overall Feelings:	Awful	Not Good	OK	Great	Awesome
Energy:	😣	😐	🙂	😁	😍
Nutrition:	😣	😐	🙂	😁	😍
Exercise:	😣	😐	🙂	😁	😍

Sleep Time:...............   Weight AM:...............   Weight AM:...............

Week Of:................................

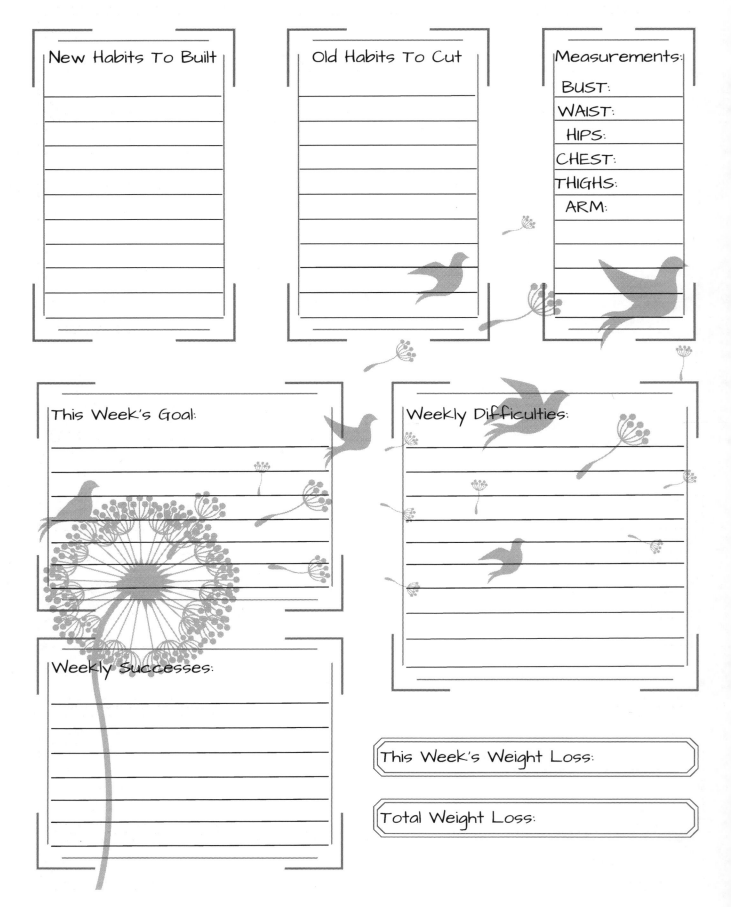

New Habits To Built

Old Habits To Cut

Measurements:
BUST:

WAIST:

HIPS:

CHEST:

THIGHS:

ARM:

This Week's Goal:

Weekly Difficulties:

Weekly Successes:

This Week's Weight Loss:

Total Weight Loss:

DATE...................................

Fasting Day? Yes No   Feeding Window: 2 4 6 8 10 12

Meals:	Time:	Calories:

Water Intake: 🥛 🥛 🥛 🥛 🥛 🥛 🥛 🥛 🥛 🥛   Supplements: 💊 💊 💊

Exercise	Time/Distance/Steps/Sets	Calories/Goal Achieved?

My Notes:
_____
_____
_____

Overall Feelings:	Awful	Not Good	OK	Great	Awesome
Energy:	😖	😐	🙂	😁	😍
Nutrition:	😖	😐	🙂	😁	😍
Exercise:	😖	😐	🙂	😁	😍

Sleep Time:............   Weight AM:..............   Weight AM:..............

DATE................................

Fasting Day? Yes No   Feeding Window: 2 4 6 8 10 12

Meals:		Time:	Calories:

Water Intake: 🥛🥛🥛🥛🥛🥛🥛🥛🥛🥛   Supplements: 💊💊💊

Exercise	Time/Distance/Steps/Sets	Calories/Goal Achieved?

My Notes:
_____
_____
_____

Overall Feelings:	Awful	Not Good	OK	Great	Awesome
Energy:	😖	😐	🙂	😃	😍
Nutrition:	😖	😐	🙂	😃	😍
Exercise:	😖	😐	🙂	😃	😍

Sleep Time:..............   Weight AM:..............   Weight AM:..............

DATE..........................

Fasting Day? Yes No   Feeding Window: 2 4 6 8 10 12

Meals:	Time:	Calories:

Water Intake: ☐ ☐ ☐ ☐ ☐ ☐ ☐ ☐ ☐ ☐   Supplements: ◌ ◌ ◌

Exercise	Time/Distance/Steps/Sets	Calories/Goal Achieved?

My Notes:

Overall Feelings:	Awful	Not Good	OK	Great	Awesome
Energy:	😖	😐	🙂	😁	😍
Nutrition:	😖	😐	🙂	😁	😍
Exercise:	😖	😐	🙂	😁	😍

Sleep Time:..............   Weight AM:..............   Weight AM:..............

DATE......................................

Fasting Day? Yes No   Feeding Window: 2 4 6 8 10 12

Meals:	Time:	Calories:

Water Intake: 🥤🥤🥤🥤🥤🥤🥤🥤🥤🥤 Supplements: 💊💊💊

Exercise	Time/Distance/Steps/Sets	Calories/Goal Achieved?

My Notes:

Overall Feelings:	Awful	Not Good	OK	Great	Awesome
Energy:					
Nutrition:					
Exercise:					

Sleep Time:...............   Weight AM:...............   Weight AM:...............

DATE.............................

Fasting Day? Yes No   Feeding Window: 2 4 6 8 10 12

Meals:		Time:	Calories:

Water Intake: [ ] [ ] [ ] [ ] [ ] [ ] [ ] [ ] [ ] [ ]   Supplements: ⊘ ⊘ ⊘

Exercise	Time/Distance/Steps/Sets	Calories/Goal Achieved?

My Notes:
_____
_____
_____

Overall Feelings:	Awful	Not Good	OK	Great	Awesome
Energy:	😖	😐	🙂	😁	😍
Nutrition:	😖	😐	🙂	😁	😍
Exercise:	😖	😐	🙂	😁	😍

Sleep Time:...........   Weight AM:...........   Weight AM:...........

DATE...

Fasting Day? Yes No   Feeding Window: 2 4 6 8 10 12

Meals:	Time:	Calories:

Water Intake: 🥛🥛🥛🥛🥛🥛🥛🥛🥛🥛   Supplements: 💊 💊 💊

Exercise	Time/Distance/Steps/Sets	Calories/Goal Achieved?

My Notes:
_____
_____
_____

Overall Feelings:	Awful	Not Good	OK	Great	Awesome
Energy:	😖	😐	🙂	😁	😍
Nutrition:	😖	😐	🙂	😁	😍
Exercise:	😖	😐	🙂	😁	😍

Sleep Time:...............   Weight AM:...............   Weight AM:...............

DATE..........................

Fasting Day? Yes No   Feeding Window: 2 4 6 8 10 12

Meals:	Time:	Calories:

Water Intake: ▯ ▯ ▯ ▯ ▯ ▯ ▯ ▯ ▯ ▯   Supplements: ⬭ ⬭ ⬭

Exercise	Time/Distance/Steps/Sets	Calories/Goal Achieved?

My Notes:

Overall Feelings:	Awful	Not Good	OK	Great	Awesome
Energy:	😖	😐	🙂	😁	😍
Nutrition:	😖	😐	🙂	😁	😍
Exercise:	😖	😐	🙂	😁	😍

Sleep Time:..............   Weight AM:..............   Weight AM:..............

Week Of:.............................

New Habits To Built

_____
_____
_____
_____
_____
_____
_____
_____
_____

Old Habits To Cut

_____
_____
_____
_____
_____
_____
_____
_____

Measurements:

BUST:
WAIST:
HIPS:
CHEST:
THIGHS:
ARM:

This Week's Goal:

_____
_____
_____
_____
_____
_____

Weekly Difficulties:

_____
_____
_____
_____
_____
_____
_____
_____
_____

Weekly Successes:

_____
_____
_____
_____
_____
_____
_____
_____

This Week's Weight Loss:

Total Weight Loss:

DATE..

Fasting Day? Yes No   Feeding Window: 2 4 6 8 10 12

Meals:		Time:	Calories:

Water Intake: 🥛🥛🥛🥛🥛🥛🥛🥛🥛🥛   Supplements: 💊💊💊

Exercise	Time/Distance/Steps/Sets	Calories/Goal Achieved?

My Notes:

Overall Feelings:	Awful	Not Good	OK	Great	Awesome
Energy:	😖	😐	🙂	😁	😍
Nutrition:	😖	😐	🙂	😁	😍
Exercise:	😖	😐	🙂	😁	😍

Sleep Time:..................   Weight AM:..................   Weight AM:..................

DATE........................

Fasting Day? Yes No   Feeding Window: 2 4 6 8 10 12

Meals:	Time:	Calories:

Water Intake: ☐ ☐ ☐ ☐ ☐ ☐ ☐ ☐ ☐ ☐   Supplements: ◌ ◌ ◌

Exercise	Time/Distance/Steps/Sets	Calories/Goal Achieved?

My Notes:
_____
_____
_____

Overall Feelings:	Awful	Not Good	OK	Great	Awesome
Energy:	😖	😐	🙂	😁	😊
Nutrition:	😖	😐	🙂	😁	😊
Exercise:	😖	😐	🙂	😁	😊

Sleep Time:...............   Weight AM:...............   Weight AM:...............

DATE......................................

Fasting Day? Yes No   Feeding Window: 2 4 6 8 10 12

Meals:		Time:	Calories:

Water Intake: 🥛🥛🥛🥛🥛🥛🥛🥛🥛🥛   Supplements: 💊💊💊

Exercise	Time/Distance/Steps/Sets	Calories/Goal Achieved?

My Notes:
_____
_____
_____

Overall Feelings:	Awful	Not Good	OK	Great	Awesome
Energy:	😖	😐	🙂	😁	😍
Nutrition:	😖	😐	🙂	😁	😍
Exercise:	😖	😐	🙂	😁	😍

Sleep Time:...............   Weight AM:...............   Weight AM:...............

DATE.............................

Fasting Day? Yes No   Feeding Window: 2 4 6 8 10 12

Meals:		Time:	Calories:

Water Intake: [glasses]   Supplements: [pills]

Exercise	Time/Distance/Steps/Sets	Calories/Goal Achieved?

My Notes:
_____
_____
_____

Overall Feelings:	Awful	Not Good	OK	Great	Awesome
Energy:	😖	😐	🙂	😁	😍
Nutrition:	😖	😐	🙂	😁	😍
Exercise:	😖	😐	🙂	😁	😍

Sleep Time:.............   Weight AM:.............   Weight AM:.............

DATE.................................

Fasting Day? Yes No   Feeding Window: 2 4 6 8 10 12

Meals:		Time:	Calories:

Water Intake: 🥛🥛🥛🥛🥛🥛🥛🥛🥛🥛   Supplements: 💊💊💊

Exercise	Time/Distance/Steps/Sets	Calories/Goal Achieved?

My Notes:

Overall Feelings:	Awful	Not Good	OK	Great	Awesome
Energy:	😖	😐	🙂	😁	😍
Nutrition:	😖	😐	🙂	😁	😍
Exercise:	😖	😐	🙂	😁	😍

Sleep Time:.............   Weight AM:.............   Weight AM:.............

DATE..

Fasting Day? Yes No   Feeding Window: 2 4 6 8 10 12

Meals:		Time:	Calories:

Water Intake: ▢ ▢ ▢ ▢ ▢ ▢ ▢ ▢ ▢ ▢   Supplements: ⬭ ⬭ ⬭

Exercise	Time/Distance/Steps/Sets	Calories/Goal Achieved?

My Notes:
_____
_____
_____

Overall Feelings:	Awful	Not Good	OK	Great	Awesome
Energy:	😖	😐	🙂	😁	😊
Nutrition:	😖	😐	🙂	😁	😊
Exercise:	😖	😐	🙂	😁	😊

Sleep Time:...............   Weight AM:...............   Weight AM:...............

DATE.................................

Fasting Day? Yes No   Feeding Window: 2 4 6 8 10 12

Meals:	Time:	Calories:

Water Intake: 🥛🥛🥛🥛🥛🥛🥛🥛🥛🥛 Supplements: 💊 💊 💊

Exercise	Time/Distance/Steps/Sets	Calories/Goal Achieved?

My Notes:

Overall Feelings:	Awful	Not Good	OK	Great	Awesome
Energy:	😖	😐	🙂	😁	😍
Nutrition:	😖	😐	🙂	😁	😍
Exercise:	😖	😐	🙂	😁	😍

Sleep Time:..............   Weight AM:..............   Weight AM:..............

Week Of:_____

New Habits To Built

Old Habits To Cut

Measurements:
BUST:

WAIST:

HIPS:

CHEST:

THIGHS:

ARM:

This Week's Goal:

Weekly Difficulties:

Weekly Successes:

This Week's Weight Loss:

Total Weight Loss:

DATE..

Fasting Day? Yes No   Feeding Window: 2 4 6 8 10 12

Meals:		Time:	Calories:

Water Intake: ⊔⊔⊔⊔⊔⊔⊔⊔⊔   Supplements: ⬭⬭⬭

Exercise	Time/Distance/Steps/Sets	Calories/Goal Achieved?

My Notes:
_____
_____
_____

Overall Feelings:	Awful	Not Good	OK	Great	Awesome
Energy:	😣	😐	🙂	😁	😊
Nutrition:	😣	😐	🙂	😁	😊
Exercise:	😣	😐	🙂	😁	😊

Sleep Time:............   Weight AM:............   Weight AM:............

DATE.........................

Fasting Day? Yes No   Feeding Window: 2 4 6 8 10 12

Meals:		Time:	Calories:

Water Intake: 🥛🥛🥛🥛🥛🥛🥛🥛🥛🥛   Supplements: 💊 💊 💊

Exercise	Time/Distance/Steps/Sets	Calories/Goal Achieved?

My Notes:

Overall Feelings:	Awful	Not Good	OK	Great	Awesome
Energy:	😣	😐	🙂	😁	😍
Nutrition:	😣	😐	🙂	😁	😍
Exercise:	😣	😐	🙂	😁	😍

Sleep Time:..............   Weight AM:...............   Weight AM:...............

DATE............................

Fasting Day? Yes No   Feeding Window: 2 4 6 8 10 12

Meals:	Time:	Calories:

Water Intake: ☐ ☐ ☐ ☐ ☐ ☐ ☐ ☐ ☐ ☐   Supplements: ◯ ◯ ◯

Exercise	Time/Distance/Steps/Sets	Calories/Goal Achieved?

My Notes:
_____
_____
_____
_____

Overall Feelings:	Awful	Not Good	OK	Great	Awesome
Energy:	😖	😐	🙂	😁	😍
Nutrition:	😖	😐	🙂	😁	😍
Exercise:	😖	😐	🙂	😁	😍

Sleep Time:............   Weight AM:............   Weight AM:............

DATE..................................

Fasting Day? Yes No   Feeding Window: 2 4 6 8 10 12

Meals:		Time:	Calories:

Water Intake: 🥛🥛🥛🥛🥛🥛🥛🥛🥛🥛   Supplements: 💊💊💊

Exercise	Time/Distance/Steps/Sets	Calories/Goal Achieved?

My Notes:
_____
_____
_____

Overall Feelings:	Awful	Not Good	OK	Great	Awesome
Energy:	😖	😐	🙂	😁	😊
Nutrition:	😖	😐	🙂	😁	😊
Exercise:	😖	😐	🙂	😁	😊

Sleep Time:...............   Weight AM:...............   Weight AM:...............

DATE................................

Fasting Day? Yes No   Feeding Window: 2 4 6 8 10 12

Meals:		Time:	Calories:

Water Intake: 🥛🥛🥛🥛🥛🥛🥛🥛🥛🥛   Supplements: 💊💊💊

Exercise	Time/Distance/Steps/Sets	Calories/Goal Achieved?

My Notes:

Overall Feelings:	Awful	Not Good	OK	Great	Awesome
Energy:	😣	😐	🙂	😁	😍
Nutrition:	😣	😐	🙂	😁	😍
Exercise:	😣	😐	🙂	😁	😍

Sleep Time:...............   Weight AM:...............   Weight AM:...............

DATE...................................

Fasting Day? Yes No   Feeding Window: 2 4 6 8 10 12

Meals:		Time:	Calories:

Water Intake: 🥛🥛🥛🥛🥛🥛🥛🥛🥛🥛   Supplements: 💊💊💊

Exercise	Time/Distance/Steps/Sets	Calories/Goal Achieved?

My Notes:

Overall Feelings:	Awful	Not Good	OK	Great	Awesome
Energy:	😖	😐	🙂	😁	😊
Nutrition:	😖	😐	🙂	😁	😊
Exercise:	😖	😐	🙂	😁	😊

Sleep Time:...............   Weight AM:...............   Weight AM:...............

DATE.............................

Fasting Day? Yes No   Feeding Window: 2 4 6 8 10 12

Meals:	Time:	Calories:

Water Intake: 🥛🥛🥛🥛🥛🥛🥛🥛🥛🥛   Supplements: ⬭⬭⬭

Exercise	Time/Distance/Steps/Sets	Calories/Goal Achieved?

My Notes:
_____
_____
_____

Overall Feelings:	Awful	Not Good	OK	Great	Awesome
Energy:	😖	😐	🙂	😁	😍
Nutrition:	😖	😐	🙂	😁	😍
Exercise:	😖	😐	🙂	😁	😍

Sleep Time:...................   Weight AM:...................   Weight AM:...................

Week Of:......................

New Habits To Built

Old Habits To Cut

Measurements:
BUST:
WAIST:
HIPS:
CHEST:
THIGHS:
ARM:

This Week's Goal:

Weekly Difficulties:

Weekly Successes:

This Week's Weight Loss:

Total Weight Loss:

DATE.........................

Meals:		Time:	Calories:

Water Intake: ▯ ▯ ▯ ▯ ▯ ▯ ▯ ▯ ▯ ▯   Supplements: ⬭ ⬭ ⬭

Exercise	Time/Distance/Steps/Sets	Calories/Goal Achieved?

My Notes:
_____
_____
_____

Overall Feelings:	Awful	Not Good	OK	Great	Awesome
Energy:	😖	😐	🙂	😁	😍
Nutrition:	😖	😐	🙂	😁	😍
Exercise:	😖	😐	🙂	😁	😍

Sleep Time:................   Weight AM:................   Weight AM:................

DATE.............................

Fasting Day? Yes No   Feeding Window: 2 4 6 8 10 12

Meals:	Time:	Calories:

Water Intake: ⬜⬜⬜⬜⬜⬜⬜⬜⬜⬜   Supplements: 💊💊💊

Exercise	Time/Distance/Steps/Sets	Calories/Goal Achieved?

My Notes:
_____
_____
_____

Overall Feelings:	Awful	Not Good	OK	Great	Awesome
Energy:	😖	😐	🙂	😁	🥰
Nutrition:	😖	😐	🙂	😁	🥰
Exercise:	😖	😐	🙂	😁	🥰

Sleep Time:.............   Weight AM:.............   Weight AM:.............

DATE...

Fasting Day? Yes No   Feeding Window: 2 4 6 8 10 12

Meals:		Time:	Calories:

Water Intake: ⬜⬜⬜⬜⬜⬜⬜⬜⬜⬜   Supplements: ⬭⬭⬭

Exercise	Time/Distance/Steps/Sets	Calories/Goal Achieved?

My Notes:
_____
_____
_____

Overall Feelings:	Awful	Not Good	OK	Great	Awesome
Energy:	😖	😐	🙂	😁	😍
Nutrition:	😖	😐	🙂	😁	😍
Exercise:	😖	😐	🙂	😁	😍

Sleep Time:...............   Weight AM:...............   Weight AM:...............

DATE............................

Fasting Day? Yes No   Feeding Window: 2 4 6 8 10 12

Meals:		Time:	Calories:

Water Intake: 🥛🥛🥛🥛🥛🥛🥛🥛🥛🥛   Supplements: 💊 💊 💊

Exercise	Time/Distance/Steps/Sets	Calories/Goal Achieved?

My Notes:
_____
_____
_____

Overall Feelings:	Awful	Not Good	OK	Great	Awesome
Energy:	😖	😐	🙂	😁	🥰
Nutrition:	😖	😐	🙂	😁	🥰
Exercise:	😖	😐	🙂	😁	🥰

Sleep Time:..............   Weight AM:..............   Weight AM:..............

DATE...................................

Fasting Day? Yes No   Feeding Window: 2 4 6 8 10 12

Meals:	Time:	Calories:

Water Intake: 🥛🥛🥛🥛🥛🥛🥛🥛🥛🥛   Supplements: 💊💊💊

Exercise	Time/Distance/Steps/Sets	Calories/Goal Achieved?

My Notes:
_____
_____
_____
_____

Overall Feelings:	Awful	Not Good	OK	Great	Awesome
Energy:	😣	😐	🙂	😁	😍
Nutrition:	😣	😐	🙂	😁	😍
Exercise:	😣	😐	🙂	😁	😍

Sleep Time:..............   Weight AM:..............   Weight AM:..............

DATE..

Fasting Day? Yes No   Feeding Window: 2 4 6 8 10 12

Meals:	Time:	Calories:

Water Intake: ▯ ▯ ▯ ▯ ▯ ▯ ▯ ▯ ▯ ▯   Supplements: ⬭ ⬭ ⬭

Exercise	Time/Distance/Steps/Sets	Calories/Goal Achieved?

My Notes:
_____
_____
_____

Overall Feelings:	Awful	Not Good	OK	Great	Awesome
Energy:	😖	😐	🙂	😁	😊
Nutrition:	😖	😐	🙂	😁	😊
Exercise:	😖	😐	🙂	😁	😊

Sleep Time:...............   Weight AM:...............   Weight AM:...............

DATE..

Fasting Day? Yes No   Feeding Window: 2 4 6 8 10 12

Meals:	Time:	Calories:

Water Intake: ⬜⬜⬜⬜⬜⬜⬜⬜⬜⬜   Supplements: ⬭⬭⬭

Exercise	Time/Distance/Steps/Sets	Calories/Goal Achieved?

My Notes:
_____
_____
_____

Overall Feelings:	Awful	Not Good	OK	Great	Awesome
Energy:	😖	😐	🙂	😁	😊
Nutrition:	😖	😐	🙂	😁	😊
Exercise:	😖	😐	🙂	😁	😊

Sleep Time:...............   Weight AM:...............   Weight AM:...............

Week Of:.................................

New Habits To Built

Old Habits To Cut

Measurements:
BUST:

WAIST:

HIPS:

CHEST:

THIGHS:

ARM:

This Week's Goal:

Weekly Difficulties:

Weekly Successes:

This Week's Weight Loss:

Total Weight Loss:

DATE........................

Fasting Day? Yes No   Feeding Window: 2 4 6 8 10 12

Meals:	Time:	Calories:

Water Intake: ☐ ☐ ☐ ☐ ☐ ☐ ☐ ☐ ☐ ☐   Supplements: ⬭ ⬭ ⬭

Exercise	Time/Distance/Steps/Sets	Calories/Goal Achieved?

My Notes:
_____
_____
_____

Overall Feelings:	Awful	Not Good	OK	Great	Awesome
Energy:	😖	😐	🙂	😁	🥰
Nutrition:	😖	😐	🙂	😁	🥰
Exercise:	😖	😐	🙂	😁	🥰

Sleep Time:...............   Weight AM:...............   Weight AM:...............

DATE..

Fasting Day? Yes No   Feeding Window: 2 4 6 8 10 12

Meals:	Time:	Calories:

Water Intake: 🥛🥛🥛🥛🥛🥛🥛🥛🥛🥛   Supplements: 💊💊💊

Exercise	Time/Distance/Steps/Sets	Calories/Goal Achieved?

My Notes:
_____
_____
_____

Overall Feelings:	Awful	Not Good	OK	Great	Awesome
Energy:	😖	😐	🙂	😁	😍
Nutrition:	😖	😐	🙂	😁	😍
Exercise:	😖	😐	🙂	😁	😍

Sleep Time:............   Weight AM:............   Weight AM:............

DATE...........................

Fasting Day? Yes No   Feeding Window: 2 4 6 8 10 12

Meals:		Time:	Calories:

Water Intake: 🥛🥛🥛🥛🥛🥛🥛🥛🥛🥛   Supplements: 💊💊💊

Exercise	Time/Distance/Steps/Sets	Calories/Goal Achieved?

My Notes:
_____
_____
_____

Overall Feelings:	Awful	Not Good	OK	Great	Awesome
Energy:	😖	😐	🙂	😁	😍
Nutrition:	😖	😐	🙂	😁	😍
Exercise:	😖	😐	🙂	😁	😍

Sleep Time:..............   Weight AM:..............   Weight AM:..............

DATE.............................

Fasting Day? Yes No   Feeding Window: 2 4 6 8 10 12

Meals:	Time:	Calories:

Water Intake: ☐☐☐☐☐☐☐☐☐☐   Supplements: ○ ○ ○

Exercise	Time/Distance/Steps/Sets	Calories/Goal Achieved?

My Notes:
_____
_____
_____

Overall Feelings:	Awful	Not Good	OK	Great	Awesome
Energy:	😣	😐	🙂	😁	😍
Nutrition:	😣	😐	🙂	😁	😍
Exercise:	😣	😐	🙂	😁	😍

Sleep Time:..............   Weight AM:..............   Weight AM:..............

DATE..

Fasting Day? Yes No   Feeding Window: 2 4 6 8 10 12

Meals:		Time:	Calories:

Water Intake: 🥛🥛🥛🥛🥛🥛🥛🥛🥛🥛   Supplements: 💊💊💊

Exercise	Time/Distance/Steps/Sets	Calories/Goal Achieved?

My Notes:
_____
_____
_____

Overall Feelings:	Awful	Not Good	OK	Great	Awesome
Energy:	😣	😐	🙂	😁	😍
Nutrition:	😣	😐	🙂	😁	😍
Exercise:	😣	😐	🙂	😁	😍

Sleep Time:................   Weight AM:................   Weight AM:................

DATE...........................

Fasting Day? Yes No   Feeding Window: 2 4 6 8 10 12

Meals:		Time:	Calories:

Water Intake: 🥛🥛🥛🥛🥛🥛🥛🥛🥛🥛   Supplements: 💊💊💊

Exercise	Time/Distance/Steps/Sets	Calories/Goal Achieved?

My Notes:
_____
_____
_____

Overall Feelings:	Awful	Not Good	OK	Great	Awesome
Energy:	😖	😐	🙂	😁	😍
Nutrition:	😖	😐	🙂	😁	😍
Exercise:	😖	😐	🙂	😁	😍

Sleep Time:............   Weight AM:............   Weight AM:............

DATE..

Fasting Day? Yes No   Feeding Window: 2 4 6 8 10 12

Meals:		Time:	Calories:

Water Intake: ▢ ▢ ▢ ▢ ▢ ▢ ▢ ▢ ▢ ▢   Supplements: ⬭ ⬭ ⬭

Exercise	Time/Distance/Steps/Sets	Calories/Goal Achieved?

My Notes:

Overall Feelings:	Awful	Not Good	OK	Great	Awesome
Energy:	😖	😐	🙂	😁	😊
Nutrition:	😖	😐	🙂	😁	😊
Exercise:	😖	😐	🙂	😁	😊

Sleep Time:................   Weight AM:................   Weight AM:................

Week Of:....................................

New Habits To Built

_____
_____
_____
_____
_____
_____
_____
_____
_____

Old Habits To Cut

_____
_____
_____
_____
_____
_____
_____
_____
_____

Measurements:

BUST:
WAIST:
HIPS:
CHEST:
THIGHS:
ARM:

This Week's Goal:

_____
_____
_____
_____
_____
_____

Weekly Difficulties:

_____
_____
_____
_____
_____
_____
_____

Weekly Successes:

_____
_____
_____
_____
_____
_____
_____
_____

This Week's Weight Loss:

Total Weight Loss:

DATE................................

Fasting Day? Yes No   Feeding Window: 2 4 6 8 10 12

Meals:		Time:	Calories:

Water Intake: ▯ ▯ ▯ ▯ ▯ ▯ ▯ ▯ ▯ ▯   Supplements: ◯ ◯ ◯

Exercise	Time/Distance/Steps/Sets	Calories/Goal Achieved?

My Notes:

Overall Feelings:	Awful	Not Good	OK	Great	Awesome
Energy:					
Nutrition:					
Exercise:					

Sleep Time:................   Weight AM:................   Weight AM:................

DATE......................

Fasting Day? Yes No   Feeding Window: 2 4 6 8 10 12

Meals:		Time:	Calories:

Water Intake: 🥛🥛🥛🥛🥛🥛🥛🥛🥛🥛   Supplements: 💊💊💊

Exercise	Time/Distance/Steps/Sets	Calories/Goal Achieved?

My Notes:
_____
_____
_____

Overall Feelings:	Awful	Not Good	OK	Great	Awesome
Energy:	😖	😐	🙂	😁	😊
Nutrition:	😖	😐	🙂	😁	😊
Exercise:	😖	😐	🙂	😁	😊

Sleep Time:.............   Weight AM:.............   Weight AM:.............

DATE.............................

Fasting Day? Yes No   Feeding Window: 2 4 6 8 10 12

Meals:		Time:	Calories:

Water Intake: ⊔ ⊔ ⊔ ⊔ ⊔ ⊔ ⊔ ⊔ ⊔   Supplements: ⊘ ⊘ ⊘

Exercise	Time/Distance/Steps/Sets	Calories/Goal Achieved?

My Notes:
_____
_____
_____

Overall Feelings:	Awful	Not Good	OK	Great	Awesome
Energy:	😖	😐	🙂	😁	😍
Nutrition:	😖	😐	🙂	😁	😍
Exercise:	😖	😐	🙂	😁	😍

Sleep Time:.............   Weight AM:.............   Weight AM:.............

DATE...........................

Fasting Day? Yes No   Feeding Window: 2 4 6 8 10 12

Meals:		Time:	Calories:

Water Intake: ▭▭▭▭▭▭▭▭▭▭   Supplements: ◯ ◯ ◯

Exercise	Time/Distance/Steps/Sets	Calories/Goal Achieved?

My Notes:
_____
_____
_____

Overall Feelings:	Awful	Not Good	OK	Great	Awesome
Energy:	😖	😐	🙂	😁	😍
Nutrition:	😖	😐	🙂	😁	😍
Exercise:	😖	😐	🙂	😁	😍

Sleep Time:...............   Weight AM:...............   Weight AM:...............

DATE.............................

Fasting Day? Yes No   **Feeding Window:** 2 4 6 8 10 12

Meals:		Time:	Calories:

Water Intake: ▯ ▯ ▯ ▯ ▯ ▯ ▯ ▯ ▯ ▯   **Supplements:** ⬭ ⬭ ⬭

Exercise	Time/Distance/Steps/Sets	Calories/Goal Achieved?

My Notes:

Overall Feelings:	Awful	Not Good	OK	Great	Awesome
Energy:	😖	😐	🙂	😁	😍
Nutrition:	😖	😐	🙂	😁	😍
Exercise:	😖	😐	🙂	😁	😍

Sleep Time:...............   Weight AM:...............   Weight AM:...............

DATE.............................

Fasting Day? Yes No   Feeding Window: 2 4 6 8 10 12

Meals:		Time:	Calories:

Water Intake: 🥛🥛🥛🥛🥛🥛🥛🥛🥛🥛   Supplements: 💊💊💊

Exercise	Time/Distance/Steps/Sets	Calories/Goal Achieved?

My Notes:
_____
_____
_____

Overall Feelings:	Awful	Not Good	OK	Great	Awesome
Energy:	😣	😐	🙂	😁	🥰
Nutrition:	😣	😐	🙂	😁	🥰
Exercise:	😣	😐	🙂	😁	🥰

Sleep Time:...............   Weight AM:...............   Weight AM:...............

DATE...................................

Fasting Day? Yes No   Feeding Window: 2 4 6 8 10 12

Meals:		Time:	Calories:

Water Intake: ▯▯▯▯▯▯▯▯▯▯ Supplements: ⬭ ⬭ ⬭

Exercise	Time/Distance/Steps/Sets	Calories/Goal Achieved?

My Notes:

Overall Feelings:	Awful	Not Good	OK	Great	Awesome
Energy:	😖	😐	🙂	😁	😊
Nutrition:	😖	😐	🙂	😁	😊
Exercise:	😖	😐	🙂	😁	😊

Sleep Time:............   Weight AM:..............   Weight AM:..............

Week Of:................................

New Habits To Built

Old Habits To Cut

Measurements:
BUST:

WAIST:

HIPS:

CHEST:

THIGHS:

ARM:

This Week's Goal:

Weekly Difficulties:

Weekly Successes:

This Week's Weight Loss:

Total Weight Loss:

DATE..................................

Fasting Day? Yes No   Feeding Window: 2 4 6 8 10 12

Meals:	Time:	Calories:

Water Intake: ☐ ☐ ☐ ☐ ☐ ☐ ☐ ☐ ☐ ☐   Supplements: ◇ ◇ ◇

Exercise	Time/Distance/Steps/Sets	Calories/Goal Achieved?

My Notes:

Overall Feelings:	Awful	Not Good	OK	Great	Awesome
Energy:	😖	😐	🙂	😁	😊
Nutrition:	😖	😐	🙂	😁	😊
Exercise:	😖	😐	🙂	😁	😊

Sleep Time:...............   Weight AM:..............   Weight AM:..............

DATE............................

Fasting Day? Yes No   Feeding Window: 2 4 6 8 10 12

Meals:	Time:	Calories:

Water Intake: ⬜⬜⬜⬜⬜⬜⬜⬜⬜⬜   Supplements: ⬭⬭⬭

Exercise	Time/Distance/Steps/Sets	Calories/Goal Achieved?

My Notes:
_____
_____
_____

Overall Feelings:	Awful	Not Good	OK	Great	Awesome
Energy:	😖	😐	🙂	😁	😍
Nutrition:	😖	😐	🙂	😁	😍
Exercise:	😖	😐	🙂	😁	😍

Sleep Time:...............   Weight AM:...............   Weight AM:...............

DATE..............................

Fasting Day? Yes No   Feeding Window: 2 4 6 8 10 12

Meals:	Time:	Calories:

Water Intake: ☐ ☐ ☐ ☐ ☐ ☐ ☐ ☐ ☐   Supplements: ◯ ◯ ◯

Exercise	Time/Distance/Steps/Sets	Calories/Goal Achieved?

My Notes:

Overall Feelings:	Awful	Not Good	OK	Great	Awesome
Energy:	😖	😐	🙂	😁	😊
Nutrition:	😖	😐	🙂	😁	😊
Exercise:	😖	😐	🙂	😁	😊

Sleep Time:................   Weight AM:................   Weight AM:................

DATE...........................

Fasting Day? Yes No   Feeding Window: 2 4 6 8 10 12

Meals:		Time:	Calories:

Water Intake: [glasses]   Supplements: [pills]

Exercise	Time/Distance/Steps/Sets	Calories/Goal Achieved?

My Notes:
_____
_____
_____

Overall Feelings:	Awful	Not Good	OK	Great	Awesome
Energy:	😖	😐	🙂	😁	😊
Nutrition:	😖	😐	🙂	😁	😊
Exercise:	😖	😐	🙂	😁	😊

Sleep Time:............   Weight AM:............   Weight AM:............

DATE................................

Fasting Day? Yes No   Feeding Window: 2 4 6 8 10 12

Meals:		Time:	Calories:

Water Intake: 🥛🥛🥛🥛🥛🥛🥛🥛🥛🥛   Supplements: 💊💊💊

Exercise	Time/Distance/Steps/Sets	Calories/Goal Achieved?

My Notes:
_____
_____
_____

Overall Feelings:	Awful	Not Good	OK	Great	Awesome
Energy:	😖	😐	🙂	😁	😍
Nutrition:	😖	😐	🙂	😁	😍
Exercise:	😖	😐	🙂	😁	😍

Sleep Time:................   Weight AM:................   Weight AM:................

DATE......................................

Fasting Day? Yes No   Feeding Window: 2 4 6 8 10 12

Meals:		Time:	Calories:

Water Intake: 🥛🥛🥛🥛🥛🥛🥛🥛🥛🥛   Supplements: 💊💊💊

Exercise	Time/Distance/Steps/Sets	Calories/Goal Achieved?

My Notes:
_____
_____
_____

Overall Feelings:	Awful	Not Good	OK	Great	Awesome
Energy:	😖	😐	🙂	😁	😊
Nutrition:	😖	😐	🙂	😁	😊
Exercise:	😖	😐	🙂	😁	😊

Sleep Time:............   Weight AM:............   Weight AM:............

DATE.......................

Fasting Day? Yes No   Feeding Window: 2 4 6 8 10 12

Meals:		Time:	Calories:

Water Intake: [glasses]   Supplements: [pills]

Exercise	Time/Distance/Steps/Sets	Calories/Goal Achieved?

My Notes:

Overall Feelings:	Awful	Not Good	OK	Great	Awesome
Energy:	😖	😐	🙂	😁	😊
Nutrition:	😖	😐	🙂	😁	😊
Exercise:	😖	😐	🙂	😁	😊

Sleep Time:.............   Weight AM:.............   Weight AM:.............

Week Of:............

New Habits To Built

Old Habits To Cut

Measurements:
BUST:

WAIST:

HIPS:

CHEST:

THIGHS:

ARM:

This Week's Goal:

Weekly Difficulties:

Weekly Successes:

This Week's Weight Loss:

Total Weight Loss:

DATE..

Fasting Day? Yes No   Feeding Window: 2 4 6 8 10 12

Meals:	Time:	Calories:

Water Intake: ☐ ☐ ☐ ☐ ☐ ☐ ☐ ☐ ☐ ☐   Supplements: ⬭ ⬭ ⬭

Exercise	Time/Distance/Steps/Sets	Calories/Goal Achieved?

My Notes:

Overall Feelings:	Awful	Not Good	OK	Great	Awesome
Energy:	☹	😐	☺	😀	😍
Nutrition:	☹	😐	☺	😀	😍
Exercise:	☹	😐	☺	😀	😍

Sleep Time:............   Weight AM:...............   Weight AM:...............

DATE...........................

| Fasting Day? Yes No | | Feeding Window: 2 4 6 8 10 12 |

Meals:		Time:	Calories:

Water Intake: 🥛🥛🥛🥛🥛🥛🥛🥛🥛🥛   Supplements: 💊💊💊

Exercise	Time/Distance/Steps/Sets	Calories/Goal Achieved?

My Notes:
_____
_____
_____

Overall Feelings:	Awful	Not Good	OK	Great	Awesome
Energy:	😖	😐	🙂	😁	😍
Nutrition:	😖	😐	🙂	😁	😍
Exercise:	😖	😐	🙂	😁	😍

| Sleep Time:............ | Weight AM:............ | Weight AM:............ |

DATE................................

Fasting Day? Yes No   Feeding Window: 2 4 6 8 10 12

Meals:	Time:	Calories:

Water Intake: ▯ ▯ ▯ ▯ ▯ ▯ ▯ ▯ ▯   Supplements: ⬭ ⬭ ⬭

Exercise	Time/Distance/Steps/Sets	Calories/Goal Achieved?

My Notes:
_____
_____
_____

Overall Feelings:	Awful	Not Good	OK	Great	Awesome
Energy:	😣	😐	🙂	😁	😍
Nutrition:	😣	😐	🙂	😁	😍
Exercise:	😣	😐	🙂	😁	😍

Sleep Time:................   Weight AM:................   Weight AM:................

DATE............................

Fasting Day? Yes No   Feeding Window: 2 4 6 8 10 12

Meals:		Time:	Calories:

Water Intake: 🥛🥛🥛🥛🥛🥛🥛🥛🥛🥛   Supplements: 💊💊💊

Exercise	Time/Distance/Steps/Sets	Calories/Goal Achieved?

My Notes:
_____
_____
_____

Overall Feelings:	Awful	Not Good	OK	Great	Awesome
Energy:	😖	😐	🙂	😁	😍
Nutrition:	😖	😐	🙂	😁	😍
Exercise:	😖	😐	🙂	😁	😍

Sleep Time:..............   Weight AM:..............   Weight AM:..............

DATE...........................

Fasting Day? Yes No   Feeding Window: 2 4 6 8 10 12

Meals:	Time:	Calories:

Water Intake: ▯ ▯ ▯ ▯ ▯ ▯ ▯ ▯ ▯ ▯   Supplements: ⬭ ⬭ ⬭

Exercise	Time/Distance/Steps/Sets	Calories/Goal Achieved?

My Notes:
_____
_____
_____

Overall Feelings:	Awful	Not Good	OK	Great	Awesome
Energy:	😖	😐	🙂	😁	😍
Nutrition:	😖	😐	🙂	😁	😍
Exercise:	😖	😐	🙂	😁	😍

Sleep Time:...........   Weight AM:...........   Weight AM:...........

DATE...

Fasting Day? Yes No   Feeding Window: 2 4 6 8 10 12

Meals:		Time:	Calories:

Water Intake: 🥛🥛🥛🥛🥛🥛🥛🥛🥛🥛   Supplements: 💊💊💊

Exercise	Time/Distance/Steps/Sets	Calories/Goal Achieved?

My Notes:
_____
_____
_____

Overall Feelings:	Awful	Not Good	OK	Great	Awesome
Energy:	😖	😐	🙂	😁	🥰
Nutrition:	😖	😐	🙂	😁	🥰
Exercise:	😖	😐	🙂	😁	🥰

Sleep Time:............   Weight AM:............   Weight AM:............

DATE................................

Fasting Day? Yes No   Feeding Window: 2 4 6 8 10 12

Meals:	Time:	Calories:

Water Intake: ▢ ▢ ▢ ▢ ▢ ▢ ▢ ▢ ▢ ▢   Supplements: ⬭ ⬭ ⬭

Exercise	Time/Distance/Steps/Sets	Calories/Goal Achieved?

My Notes:
_____
_____
_____

Overall Feelings:	Awful	Not Good	OK	Great	Awesome
Energy:	😖	😐	🙂	😁	😍
Nutrition:	😖	😐	🙂	😁	😍
Exercise:	😖	😐	🙂	😁	😍

Sleep Time:................   Weight AM:................   Weight AM:................

Week Of:..................................

New Habits To Built

Old Habits To Cut

Measurements:
BUST:

WAIST:

HIPS:

CHEST:

THIGHS:

ARM:

This Week's Goal:

Weekly Difficulties:

Weekly Successes:

This Week's Weight Loss:

Total Weight Loss:

Made in United States
Orlando, FL
10 January 2025

57079450R00065